FREE

Forgive. Release. Evolve. Explore

Brandi Rae

FREE

FREE

Published by Brandi Rae Business Consulting

ISBN: 979-8-234-02737-5

FREE is brought to you, by life!

DEDICATION

It took five years to write FREE. The result of a nine-year cycle of lessons that repeated themselves as I worked my way through the encrypted messages of life lessons. Even once I acknowledged the lessons and began closing toxic cycles out of my life, it still took time to really find peace in all aspects of life. When you are one with peace, you notice how free you feel.

I would like to thank life, for lifen' me; teaching me; guiding me; and loving me.

CONTENTS

PROLOGUE

The word "free" has a definition in the dictionary; however, we individually define free based on our experience with the word. Free is untamed; it is unhinged; it is the space our inner self feels the safest. As you journey through this book, take your time. Some parts of the book may require more time to work through than others.

Some sections you may want to circle back to recurringly while proceeding with the book. Whatever you do, take your time and be patient with yourself as you explore emotions that may be tender. In this space, there is no such concept of time. There is no judgement, so be honest with yourself as you read and go through the emotions. Read the book, then go back section by section. Or work your way through, repeating sections until you are ready to proceed. Embrace your healing to set yourself free!

Without further or do, "FREE"

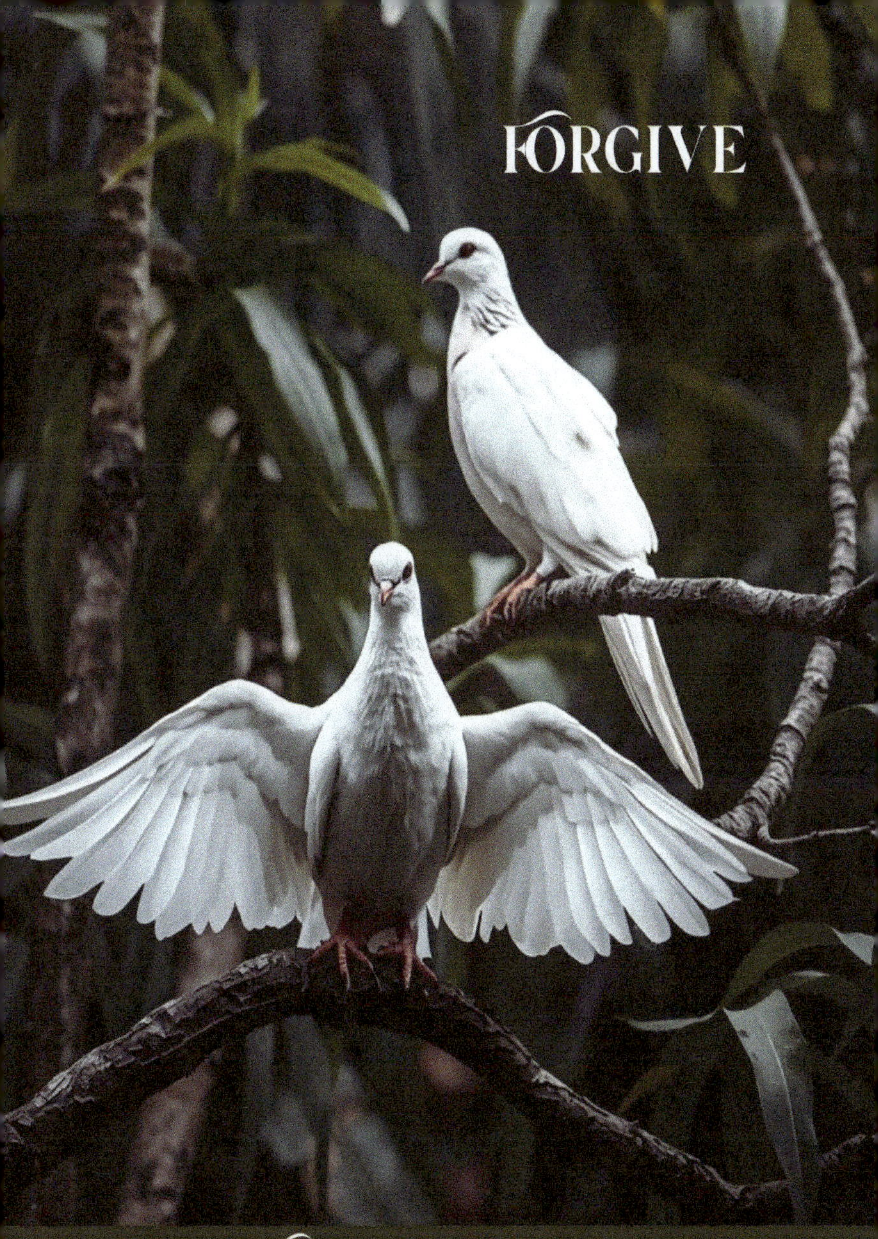

FORGIVENESS

FOSTERS PEACE

THE DOVE SYMBOLIZES RECONCILLIATION,
PEACE & NEW BEGINNINGS.

FORGIVE
HURT PEOPLE, HURT PEOPLE.

Forgiveness. One of the most challenging concepts in the healing process. The weight of our thoughts can be so heavy and dense when we feel wronged - our hearts easily become conflicted to the idea of forgiveness. Pain has a way of lingering around the subconscious as we attempt to let go of matters that left behind a scar. Yet, as challenging as forgiveness may be, understanding the definition of forgiveness is necessary to begin the healing journey.

When we allow forgiveness to break through the restraints of conflict, the weight we feel begins to lift. First, the focus of the book will be centered on forgiveness. What is forgiveness, the types of forgiveness, how to overcome the restrictions of forgiving, and understanding the balance between forgiveness and the level of access to you.

What is Forgiveness

Reflective Thought
As long as I hold on to the pain, the pain holds on to my power.

Mantra
I will take the necessary steps to face the pain and heal.

Practicing Peace
Learn how to Breathe

What is forgiveness? The overarching definition of forgiveness is to release feelings of resentment and anger when someone has offended you or caused you pain. It is much easier to say you have forgiven, than taking the steps to forgive. Forgiveness requires understanding, patience and an undetermined amount of time – and there are some offenses, some words, that simply will never be truly forgiven; instead, we use it as guidance for the future. Often, forgiveness can be mistaken for acceptance by the offender – yet acceptance embodies its own content, a separate topic. There are three different types of forgiveness – exoneration, endurance, and emancipation. You may be thinking, "wait, now there are different forms of forgiveness?" Yes, there are, as not all offenses are equal.

When we exonerate, we forgive under the understanding that the offense was genuinely an accident. There is no pattern, jealousy, or malice – instead the offense was a matter of unintentional negligence or ignorance. When we practice endurance during the forgiveness process, we accept our role in the offense that triggered the offender. Many times, triggers are unknown, but extremely provocative. An offender may react to a trigger that was never intended to create chaos; however, the response to the trigger is intentional and unfair. And finally, there is the emancipation process – where we release the connection with the offender, realizing the offense is repetitive and the pain has surpassed the boundary of acceptance.

PRACTICING PEACE

Learning how to breathe helps to defy the anxieties created when reflecting. With a straight back and still hands, allow your shoulders to drop as you prepare to take a deep breath. Next, inhale through your nose allowing air to fill your lungs and expand your belly – exhale slowly through your mouth allowing your belly to restrict as the air is released. With each exhale, drop your shoulders. Repeat this as many times as you like, but a minimum of seven times. As you do, your body will physically begin to relax. Thus, allowing your thoughts to slow down, your emotions to calm and rationalization to set in.

Daily Reflection: *Is it easy for you to forgive others?*

Daily Release: *Release a negative thought, any thought, that you are holding onto without reason.*

Exonerate

Reflective Thought

Understand the pain inflicted was without malicious intent. Accidents happen.

Mantra

I am not perfect, and I make mistakes. No one is perfect, and we all make mistakes.

Practicing Peace

Breathing and blocking out interference

Exoneration. In short, ***exonerate*** is defined as releasing from guilt and deeming innocent. One of the most unique characteristics in human nature is our ability to perceive life from different viewpoints. Our perceptions feed into how we process information; we individually gather, organize, and interpret incoming stimuli which influences our behavior.

We tend to hurt those closest to us, without intention. It may be as simple as a misunderstanding of what is said, or as big as physical harm being inflicted with no malicious intent. In such circumstances, an apology typically follows without hesitation, further reassuring the offense was an accident and allowing forgiveness to take place. On the contrary, if there is no immediate apology and offense is taken – that can make us question intent which influences rather or not we choose to forgive.

Take a moment to reflect on the situation. Even when the offense carries no malice, we naturally should give ourselves time to process our feelings and gain control over our emotions. Emotional control opens the mind to rationalize a response and properly manage our emotions. Because the time to process is undetermined, it is important to allow all the time that is needed.

PRACTICING PEACE

Now that we have learned how to relax through breathing, let's layer on blocking interference. As you begin with your breathing technique, find one sound, it may be a bird chirping, a dog barking, or water dripping. Focusing on that sound only, close your eyes and allow the sound to take you to a place of peace. As you focus on breathing and your sound, you will naturally cancel out negative thoughts. In the beginning, this can be more challenging and that is ok; overtime, it will become natural. If negative thoughts begin to seep in, redirect your thoughts and continue breathing. Meditative music can also be used to support clearing the mind.

Daily Reflection: *Is it easy to apologize when you offend others?*

Daily Release: *Release a misunderstanding that has long since been over but unnecessarily continues to linger.*

Endure

Reflective Thought
Once I take accountability for my actions, I can understand other perspectives.

Mantra
I will keep an open mind without losing site of the matter.

Practicing Peace
Breathing, Blocking & Reflecting

When life brings you lemons, you must decide what purpose the lemons serve in your life; will you be making iced tea, lemon sorbet, using as a cleaning agent? As humans, being accountable is an essential part of interacting with one another. When we choose the route of ***endurance*** when forgiving, at some point you have accepted your role in the matter, allowing you to move forward with maintaining some form of relationship with the offender, even if the dynamics of the relationship alter.

Let's use a relatable example to break it down. You find yourself in an intense argument with a loved one, and they begin spewing hurtful words your way, and you are at a loss for the unsolicited behavior and how it even got to this point. Once everyone is calm, your loved one apologizes, and shares that they felt you were ignoring them when they were expressing their feelings, which resulted in them losing control and reacting impulsively out of frustration.

Rather you were ignoring the other person or that was their assumption, what is clear is they were not feeling heard by you. In that moment, taking accountability is important. "Hey, I was multitasking, and my attention was with you the entire time. I should have acknowledged you initially. However, I am deeply hurt by what was said, and your words were not acceptable."

Once you have had proper time to reflect on the incident, you now must determine what level of access the person now has to you. As essential as communication is, accountability is equally important. Taking accountability reduces the likelihood of you experiencing a cycle of guilt over your actions and allowing you to process the situation with less mental interference.

PRACTICING PEACE

Let's continue to build on our moment of peace. We practiced breathing. Breathing and blocking and now let's throw reflecting in the mix. Reflection provides space between our personal emotions and the situation. As you begin relaxing through your breaths, block all noises, and go back to the very moment when you felt wronged, hurt, or whatever respective unpleasant feeling you experienced – go back to that moment. What caused you to feel how you felt? What actions or words followed? Has this happened before? Ask yourself the questions to help arrive at a decision of where this person stands in your life. Do not rush your thoughts during reflection or rush to a decision. Allow yourself to experience each emotion that comes forward as you answer each question you ask yourself. Breathe through the emotions and let your mental guard down, so you can properly get through the experience and not band aid the situation.

Daily Reflection: *Are you able to let go of a situation when the other person has not taken accountability?*

Daily Release: *Release a guilty thought that is weighing heavy on you.*

Emancipate

Reflective Thought
Mental freedom allows space for growth.

Mantra
I will set myself free from thoughts that restrict my happiness.

Practicing Peace
Grounding & Positive Affirmations

When there is no going back, emancipation has taken place. Certain lines, once crossed, there is no crossing back. Emancipated forgiveness permanently changes the dynamics of the relationship. Now, just because the relationship is severed, that does not mean that forgiveness is not required. The emotions that were felt (and possibly lingering) are still valid and require attention.

For emotional liberation to be fulfilled, all guilt and grudges must be released within self and resolved towards the other individual. Guilt may start off light; however, the longer it sits on your conscious, the heavier it gets as it leans on you, weightless, in a very invasive manner. Guilt is resolved through taking accountability. If you find yourself circling back to a situation time and time again, questioning your actions, going over how it all played out. It is likely that there is some accountability that has not been taken on your end, interfering with you letting go of the matter – lingering in subtle subconscious guilt.

Similarly, grudges add unnecessary mental weight and can interfere with how you show up. Let's use a scenario, say you don't want to be in the same room as the person with whom you are holding the grudge. Now every time there is an event, your decision to go is influenced by another's presence. Now this is only one example; the point being, holding a grudge is an attack on self. Grudges are like long chains, that allow you to go far but never allow you to get away – you are chained down by the thought. The way to escape is to remove yourself from the chain and walk away. Don't overthink releasing a grudge.

Daily Reflection: *Have you ever let go of something mentally and physically felt the weight lift?*

Daily Release: *Release a grudge – no matter how big or small. It can be recent or dating back to childhood. Dig deeper and let go of as many grudges as you can. Life will be, what life will be.*

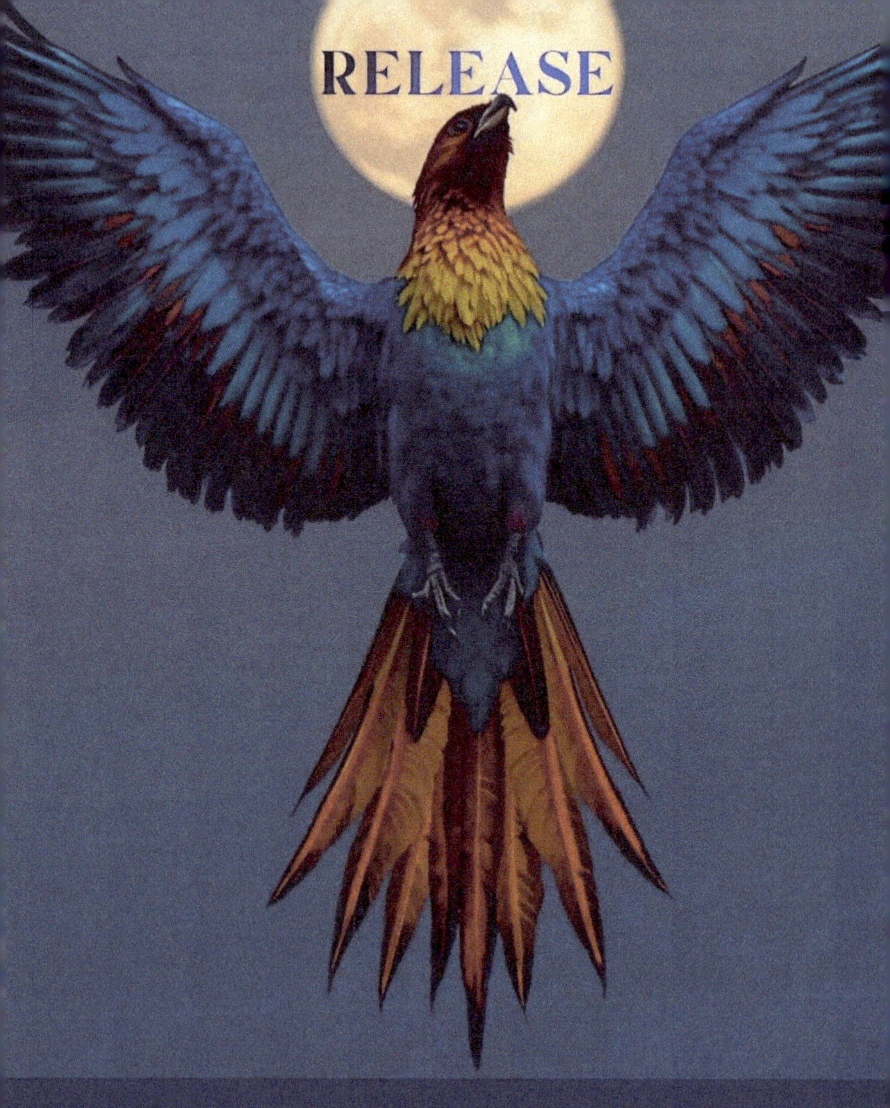

HEAD HIGH TO THE SKY,

WITH PHOENIX EYES.

THE PHOENIX SYMBOLIZES PERSONAL RENEWAL BY LETTING GO OF OUTDATED, LIMITING BELIEFS.

RELEASE

Make it make sense, and if it no longer does, let it go.

Space is infinite, however, that does not mean that space is not filled with miscellaneous matter that serves no purpose other than aimlessly orbiting through space. The same goes for our mental and physical space. Once an idea, a place, a relationship, a job, a way of life no longer serves purpose to the current version of you, it must be released for the right alignment with the new version of you. When we are young, our feet grow continuously, until one day, they stop growing. But during this drawn outgrowth period, we are forced to purchase larger shoes to accommodate the growth. No matter how comfy or how connected you may have been to a pair of shoes, you had to let them go at some point. Then we reach late teens or early adulthood, and our feet pretty much plateau in growth. Now you can rock those comfy shoes – you can rock them until the soles fall off and keep stepping. You don't even realize that the shoe is so worn down, it is no longer comfortable, but you are used to it now. You've normalized discomfort and replaced reality with familiarity. The shoes no longer serve their purpose of comfort and security.

The Fear of Forgiving

Reflective Thought

Fear is a gateway emotion to hate, anger, resentment, anxiety – the list goes on.

Mantra

I am conquering my fear of forgiving to allow space for peace.

Moment in Peace

4 -7 - 8 then Meditate

Fear is a common roadblock that surfaces in many life situations. Often, we do not realize that we lead with fear over confidence in most situations. Understanding how fear influences our mind, our motives, the way we operate, and our better judgement is the first step to overcoming the fear of rather or not, we choose to forgive.

What makes it hard to forgive? The thought that someone will get away with hurting you or diminishing your character. The assumption that if you do not hold on to the issue, you lose power or you lose control. The truth is, you are powerless if someone can dictate your emotions, thoughts, and even the way you process information. When we forgive, we release weight. We remove the stagnant and stale energy allowing space for growth and room for energy to support the growth.

Imagine a five-pound weight added around your waist every time you held on to a situation out of fear of forgiving. How long would you be able to endure the weight before breaking down? How strong will you have to be to carry around burdens from the past that are weighing you down? It would not be long before you completely break, become disgruntled, and adapt an overall sense of anger toward life. On the flip side, forgiving those who have wronged you allows you to focus on YOU and what brings YOU joy, peace, and fulfillment.

So why does forgiveness strike fear? Because we become vulnerable during an already complex mental state. There is the fear of not being in control of your emotions, words, thoughts. The uncertainty around how others may react or respond both in the present time and the future. If I forgive this person, will they do this to me again? What if there is more to the story and I forgive them, but under false pretense? Any number of questions can cross your mind when considering forgiving someone, but those curiosities, uncertainties, endless thoughts poke at your securities making you raise your guard out of fear.

In essence, the fear stems from overthinking. If we take the time to reflect on the situation. Acknowledge the feelings that were experienced at the time and don't forget about the lingering emotions that interrupt your thoughts from time to time. Be present in the decision that you are making without hiding from discomfort.

MOMENT IN PEACE

Let's wrap up this section with our moment of peace. As we continue this journey, we are ready to layer on a unique breathing technique before meditating. The 4-7-8 breathing technique is something I use when I feel my emotions and thoughts are coming in hot. Before the internal chaos escalates, I inhale for four seconds, hold that breath for seven seconds, and release it over eight seconds. I repeat it until I feel my shoulders drop with ease and I feel a peaceful calm wrapping around me, like a blanket, comforting me. After you have come to a comfortable space, ease into a meditation session.

NOTE: The number of seconds you hold your breath during the 4-7-8 breathing exercise should be based on what feels best for you and your health.

Daily Reflection: *How often do you find yourself hoping you will be forgiven?*

Daily Release: *Release the fear of vulnerability. Has the fear of being vulnerable consumed you to the point that you are unable to forgive and move beyond a situation. Is there fear around the person getting the best of you?*

Forgiving Yourself

Reflective Thought

Perfection is an illusion; but I am real. My feelings are valid.

Mantra

I give myself permission to have compassion for myself.

Moment of Peace

Releasing guilt as you forgive yourself

There, in the deceitful heart of illusion, lies perfection. Perfection has a special glow, bringing about a radiant mental image, a feeling of eminence. Perfection can give such an immense high, that your world feels shattered when reality sets in and eminence is replaced with emotions. No matter which end of the stick you're at, offender or the one being offended – releasing burdens of guilt is required for personal growth. For moving forward and allowing space for self-compassion.

Mistakes are a key aspect in learning as you travel through life's journey. Mistakes foster growth and redefine self-image. Some mistakes can leave a feeling of burden from the mental and emotional load of guilt. Burdens are blockers, prohibiting your ability to see beyond shame. Burdens bring doubt and insecurities as you stumble through the land of going back in time, distancing yourself further from your future. Guilt, burdens, shame – must all be released for you to continue your journey.

Let's transform this mental load to a physical load to create a relatable concept. Say you have a backpack and you set off for a walk to meet your health goal. Let's say this is the final stretch of your health journey to accomplish your goals. Now, in that backpack, there is a rock for every burden you are carrying with you on this journey – weight that has attached to you mentally and starting to impact you physically. How long before you start to slow down from exhaustion? How long before the weight becomes unbearable? How long before your body begins to break down? Your mental and physical health balances off one another; they work hand in hand, so both are equally important to manage.

The anguish of guilt is a mental weight – holding your mind hostage. Restricting you from your fullest physical potential. Irregular or inconsistent breathing. Impaired nervous system. Headaches. Unexplained aches and pains. Obesity. Anorexia. High blood pressure. Sleepless nights that result in low energy. The list goes on, but I am sure the point has been made. Your mental and physical health are intertwined. Once you remove the backpack and walk away, there is a sense of relief encouraging you to get as far away from the weight, allowing space for healing. The baggage of burdens will surely slow you down. Be forgiving of yourself. Be gentle with yourself. Find a safe place within you. Liberate your emotions from your burdens.

MOMENT OF PEACE

Now, let's practice some peace! In a quiet place, reflect on a situation that you still hold guilt over. Allow yourself to be present in the moment, no matter the feelings that arise as you recall the situation. As you breathe in, tell yourself, "I am enough." As you exhale, tell yourself, "I release all burdens and I forgive myself."

Daily Reflection: *Have you ever repeatedly reflected on a situation and felt worse every time you thought about it? Now ask yourself, does the guilt you are carrying change what happened? Does guilt do anything for your personal growth in moving forward? If the answer to the last two questions is, "no" – release the guilt. It will not change anything.*

Daily Release: *Release the backpack. Do not try and unload it. Release it.*

The Reality of Forgiveness

Reflective Thought
Forgiveness is you choosing peace & freedom.

Mantra
It's my personal choice to choose peace and return unwanted energy to the sender.

Moment of Peace
Go for a walk and let your mind wander

The reality of forgiveness is that it isn't easy. There is a phrase "Water under the bridge" that symbolizes the flow of water that has passed and that is that. The challenge in forgiving is the memory of the offence and the inability to forget how you felt in the situation. There is a high likelihood of reliving emotions, thoughts, or the outcome until you have fully healed. Yet in life, it is not that simple to walk away from an experience that includes trauma. It is ok to be vulnerable as your feelings will likely fluctuate until the peace is fully restored.

Establishing peace is essential to avoid being triggered in the future. Peace allows your emotions to remain stable when faced with similar situations that provoke reliving the memory or encountering the offender. It is important to understand that peace helps control your emotional responses to triggers – this does not mean triggers will not occur. Now let's take a moment to reflect on what brought about the need to forgive. In this moment, what are your expectations for the future? What are the dynamics of this relationship moving forward? Next to establishing peace, it is crucial to conclude how you wish to proceed with the offender. Are you able to be cordial in public/private places? Is it best to never come into contact? Do you share any responsibilities that require a direct form of communication. Once you arrive at the most appropriate dynamic, that is in line with maintaining peace- proceed with setting boundaries. Congrats, you have created a bridge of unity between forgiveness and peace.

MOMENT OF PEACE

Embrace a moment of peace with nature by going for a walk. If possible, connect in nature or outdoors. If not, that is ok, stroll around your home. The purpose behind the movement is to allow your mind to wander, as you wander and allow yourself to tap in with self. As you move, notice the thoughts that are coming to the surface. Did you go straight to tasks on a "to do" list. Or do you drift off into the future? Allow your mind to run free, from topic to topic. Any negative thoughts that come into play, reject them. You do not own those thoughts, so don't entertain them.

Daily Reflection: *Do you start with forgiving yourself?*

Daily Release: *Release the negative thoughts of self.*

Let Your Emotions Run Wild

Reflective Thought

Even a waterfall has a period of dormancy – but when it flows, it does so naturally.

Mantra

As my emotions flow out, I am releasing. I am healing.

Moment of Peace

Releasing Your Inner Emotions

Time to release. Forgiveness is the beginning of a journey as we learn to release what has lost its influence over us. Releasing what no longer adds to our individual greatness, lightens the surrounding energy and attracts positivity. When we let go, space opens for what is to come next. New paths of growth began to present themselves. Think of a plant, once it outgrows its pot, new growth slows down tremendously and growth may stagnate altogether. Once the plant is repotted, growth can take place once more.

Some matters are more complex. Let's imagine a room filled with boxes. Some boxes are empty; some have rubbish contents; others have property that does not belong to you. What value do the boxes hold? First, you must sort through the boxes and see what should remain and what should be returned to the rightful owner. Now purge the rest! Remove the misplaced boxes and fill the room with your desires – make it a safe place where you can thrive, have peace, be yourself. The analogies can go on, but safe to say, the essence of releasing brings in more than what was released.

Releasing, however, is dependent upon forgiving. It is challenging to release what is unresolved. Human nature often seeks closure. Think of leaving a job or school, you may be asked to participate in an exit survey. When you end a subscription, the vendor wants to know, "why?" As a relationship ends, there is desire to understand or attempt to understand, the true cause. If the door is still open, thoughts, emotions, actions, etc. will continue to flow inward disrupting the true, full release. In some cases, you will have to accept no closure, as closure – knowing whatever the reason the relations or situation served its purpose in your journey.

MOMENT OF PEACE

Now let's take the time to do some inner work, releasing in a way that is right for you. That may be screaming in a pillow. Crying in the shower and allowing the water to wash away the tears and unwanted energy. Listening to your favorite playlist. I personally love connecting in nature and I love catching windy days and going for a slow stroll in my neighborhood, allowing the wind to lead me. Mother nature is so powerful, being outside allows me to release into a space large enough and powerful enough to absorb all I must release.

Daily Reflection: *What does release look like to you?*

Daily Release: *Release something physical that is tied to an unpleasant memory.*

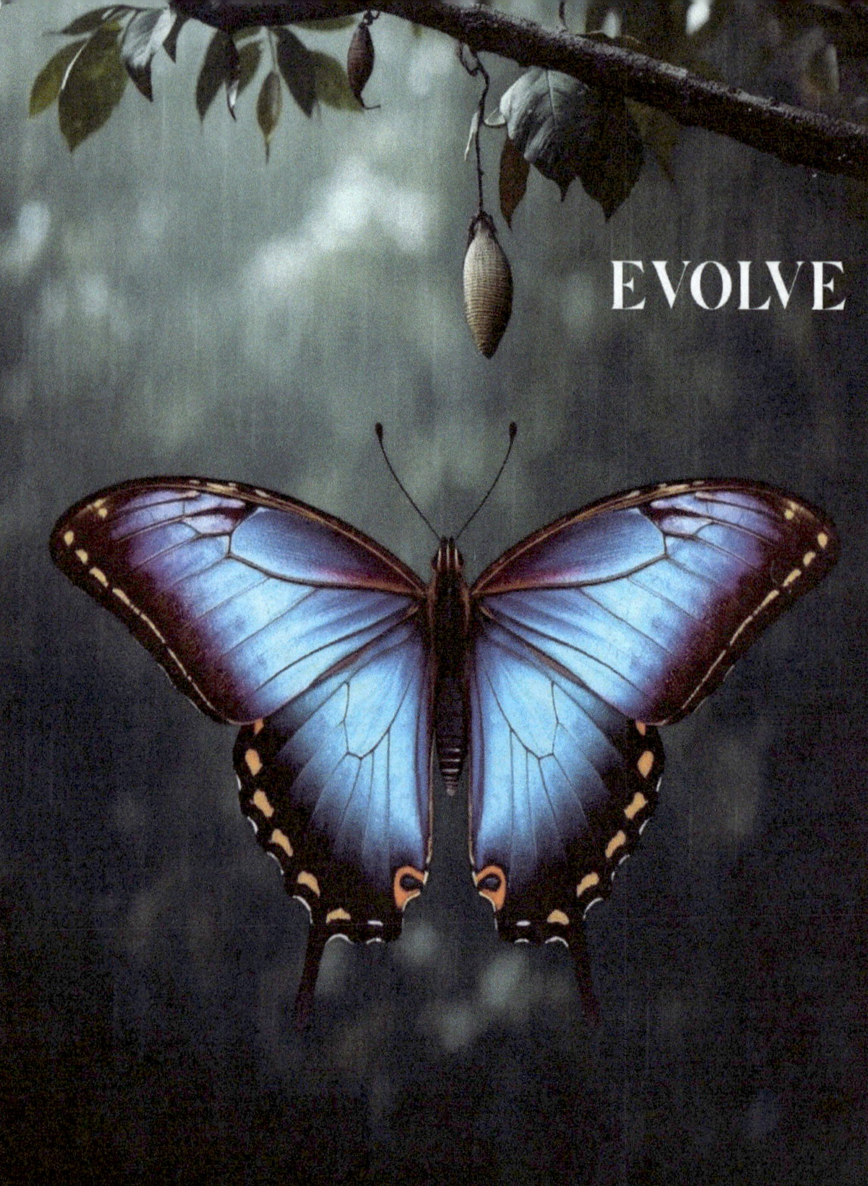

SHED YOUR COCOON

THE BUTTERFLY SYMBOLIZES PERSONAL GROWTH AND REBIRTH THROUGH TRANSFORMATION.

THE INNER YOU CALLS FOR METAMORPHESIS

Who are you? Who are you in this moment? Who were you five years ago? Ten years ago? Who will you become? Growth makes evolution non optional. There is no growth without evolving. We undergo transformations as we head down our path and experiences begin to shape our existence. Our purpose. Our direction. Evolution opens doors to new opportunities that have been waiting to be approached. New interests to explore. New ways of life support a balanced sense of self. Evolution builds character and strength. It not only teaches us but gives us the knowledge to teach others. With all the power wrapped into evolution, it is not as straightforward when actually walking the walk. Evolution involves stripping most, if not all, of your comfort zones. Undergoing an ego death. Accepting that friction is all part of the process to achieve personal transformation and growth. But the moment you take the first step towards shedding what no longer belongs as part of your identity, the moment you feel the change. Now, continue to place one foot in front of the other, allowing transformation to naturally unfold.

Unbutton the Top Button

Reflective Thought

Understanding the lesson in our missteps, offers security in our next steps.

Mantra

I come as is, because I am enough.

Bring in Peace

Warm Himalayan Salt Foot Soak

Unbutton the top button. In other words, release yourself from self-imposed restrictions. Just as you are capable to button to the top, you can unbutton to release pressure. Now that you've begun to release and make space, remember to set your thoughts and expectations free from the box that enclosed them. That box is a comfort zone. Comfort breeds stagnation. Comfort comes in many shapes and sizes. It could be a relationship, a job, a way of life, habits, mentalities, thoughts – a comfort zone is just that, a space that brings you comfort. But that space is small, cramped, no breathing room, yet, so cozy and predictable.

Jog back to the miscellaneous boxes taking up space- sitting and collecting dust, stagnant. Now let's take a moment to distinguish between content and comfort. Comfort is external, people, places, habits, material items encouraging comfort and complacency. The predictability of life gives a false sense of satisfaction and the impression of happiness.

Contrary to external comfort, contentment is internal – appreciation and satisfaction of your current status, regardless of your circumstances. Contentment breeds resilience and peace within; allowing calm and stillness to encourage growth.

Comfort is stagnation; contentment is growth. Release expectations to free your thoughts from the box. Your appreciation for life and quality of life will naturally enhance when you release what doesn't belong and when you expand beyond your comfort zone.

BRING IN PEACE

When I reflect on what it means to start over, it reminds me how important it is to build a solid foundation. Let's bring in some peace by catering to our physical foundation, our feet. Rather it be in the shower, or a bath, or a foot tub – soak your feet in warm Himalayan salt water. In doing so, it helps to release toxins in the body, promote relaxation and improve circulation – amongst a host of other benefits. If possible, treat yourself to a reflexology session.

Daily Reflection: *What is a comfort zone you have been holding on to, that is holding you back from growth?*

Daily Release: *Release a comfort zone that no longer serves you, but instead, restricts you.*

Accept & Reject Insecurities

Reflective Thought
Failure is simply a lesson learned – not defeat.

Mantra
I challenge failure with success.

Bring in Peace
Laugh more often

Failure generally carries a negative connotation – but what exactly is failure? Why is failure so bad? Failure can be summarized as not achieving a goal as expected. Maybe your expectation was bias and reality was not aligned; therefore, deterring you from success. What failure is NOT, is defeat. It is a chance to reflect, regroup and recharge. You've learned a lesson, take the lesson, accept the reality of this occurrence and reject the thoughts and feelings of defeat.

The beauty in failure is that it allows you to grow in areas you once struggled, now that you have come through yet another challenge. Even if it was not to your expectation, it was necessary to build your knowledge, strengthen you, and ground your perseverance.

Now you are more powerful than ever. The moment in which failure was experienced is now in the past. That chapter has ended, for some, the book has ended. Gently tuck the book away, not as if forgotten and no need to re-read the story- but a casual glance at the neatly tucked book- shall serve as a gentle reminder of the lesson learned.

Making mistakes and failing is all part of the process of building and continued growth. Making the same mistakes repeatedly is different; there is intention in repetition and indicates the lesson has not been learned. It can also be self-sabotaging by continuing a cycle yet anticipating change, without trying a new approach. In conclusion, failure is not negative; Mistakes are meant to happen; lessons foster growth. What matters is how you handle the lessons brought to you. How do you use it as a ladder to success versus a shovel to dig yourself a pit, for your solo pity party.

BRING IN PEACE

Laughter cuts through negativity. Bring in peace and counter negativity with laughter. Laugh frequently, find moments in the day and reflect on memories that bring joy and laughter and release thoughts of insecurities. Laugher creates space for happiness to grow. As happiness spreads, your general mood increases, your perspectives expand, your insecurities begin to fade away because you've accepted failure as a lesson and did not allow it to stop you. You get the last laugh – not failure.

Daily Reflection: *Do you sit in a mental pit when failure comes your way? Or do you use failure as a steppingstone?*

Daily Release: *Release a thought that has caused a reoccurring fear of failure and created invisible barriers.*

Slow Down

Reflective Thought

I am deliberately taking my leisure time to process my thoughts; align my words with actions and understand my emotions.

Mantra

I find peace in stillness.

Bring in Peace

Resetting your energy through stillness

Peace is the blanket, the comfort, the safe place for your nervous system. Imagine being wrapped in a blanket, fireplace blazing on a winter night and you find that cozy place and that sense of calm envelops your soul. Now, out of nowhere, you have to use the restroom, forcing you out of your comfort zone. No matter how hard you try or how close you come, you never get back to that original cozy place.

Constant movement, rather it be racing thoughts or physical movement is likely to disrupt peace, eventually impacting your nervous system. Slow down and give yourself space to step back and analyze your mental, emotional, physical, and financial state of being. Is there anything that does not align with you or your goals? Are you carrying what belongs to others? Is there anything that is slipping through the cracks and requires dedicated attention? Asking yourself these questions during a period of stillness helps with clarity. As the answers flow, you also fall into overall alignment.

During a moment of pause, you may question something you have been subconsciously doing or subconsciously agreeing to. The moment of reflection brings to light a decision you have to make. Do I proceed as I was? Do I proceed with caution? Do I not proceed? It is natural to layer extra details on a situation or tasks. Yet, it is equally natural to miss important details in a situation or task. Rather you are overthinking or underthinking slow down and be still. Reflect on the overall picture to bring better alignment with your reality and the decision being made. There is a misconception that life must be moving in a flash all the time. Keep-up or you'll get left behind type vibes. Get left behind. It's ok to move to a rhythmic pace suited for you. No matter how many folks can walk alongside your journey, only your footprints open the passages along your personal journey.

BRING IN PEACE

Let's bring in some peace. Stop what you are doing and sit in stillness throughout the day. Take some deep breaths to reset your energy. Coming back to center and calming your thoughts supports a healthy nervous system. Bring in peace with every breath. Choose a frequency that accommodates your lifestyle, but a minimum of three times a day is recommended. Sometimes, I catch myself shedding a few tears when I slow down. Tears of gratitude, overwhelm, laughter, pain, etc. – tears that were fighting to be released. The purpose of some tears remains unknown, but they made their way out, alongside the release of each breath. Allow stillness to bring you peace.

Daily Reflection: *How often do you acknowledge the state of your nervous system? Are YOU checking in with YOU?*

Daily Release: *Release a painful event through stillness. Allow true and honest release.*

Use Your Strong Voice

Reflective Thought
Use your voice to confirm your presence.

Mantra
I speak my truth.

Bring in Peace
Positive Affirmations

Sometimes, we mask the pain and burdens for others by giving in to a sense of guilt - self-imposed guilt. In some instances, guilt can linger into regret as if you have done something wrong, when you simply choose yourself. Reflect on the lessons that have been learned. Remind yourself that you deserve the love, the patience, and the compassion that you give to others.

Don't allow other's projections to disrupt a decision you made due to choices they made. Prepare yourself for the emotional turbulence as you juggle living beyond your shaky voice. The shaky voice that struggles with releasing guilt that never belonged. The shaky voice that gives way to your insecurities. Juggle the emotional turbulence with the shaky voice and step into your strong voice. Your strong voice that shows up with poise and calm confirmation. A voice that builds boundaries that are respected. A voice that speaks with confidence and ease. Use your strong voice and stand in the decision you made. Don't break contract with self.

BRING IN PEACE

Affirmations are real. Take some time to either write down or ponder areas where you could be more assertive and create supporting affirmations. Remember, affirmations can be simple, it does not have to be complex. One of my go to affirmations when I am not feeling heard is, "I am enough!" Simple, but does the trick. Reminding myself that I am enough automatically cloaks me with confidence. Say it enough, you begin to believe it and walk the talk!

Daily Reflection: *Does "not feeling heard" influence your confidence and how you assert your voice?*

Daily Release: *Release your insecurities verbally and replace with an affirmation.*

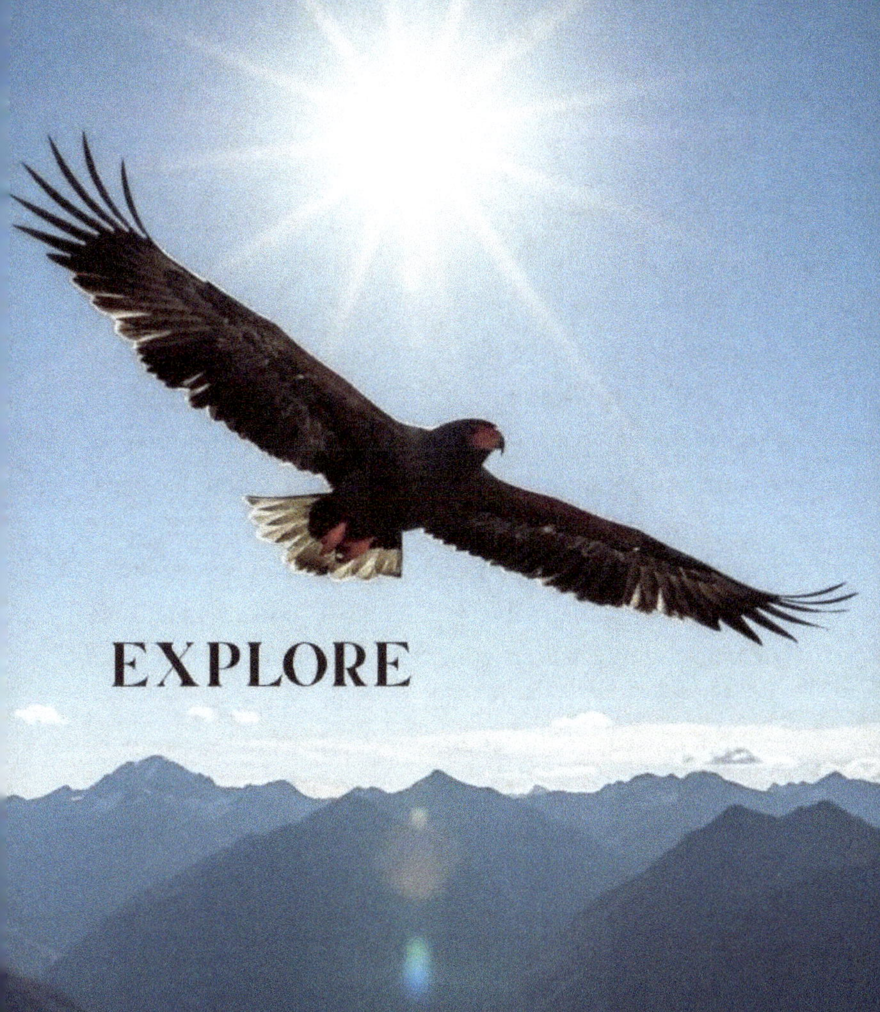

BE A FEARLESS CONQUEROR, EXPLORING LIFE FROM YOUR PERSPECTIVE

THE BATELEUR EAGLE SYMBOLIZES CONFIDENCE, OVERCOMING, AND BOUNDLESS AMBITION.

ALLOW ME TO INTRODUCE MYSELF

Who is that? You have gone from asking yourself, "who you are," to folks admiring the new you! You are at an "untouchable" place – and not in an arrogant manner, it is pure and genuine confidence. You have taken the steps and gone through the process of healing. You have reached a new sense of peace that leveled up your aura; your presence; your vibe is undeniable. You are in a place of being whole within you. Now as you explore all the world has for you and walk in your purpose, you are bound to attract the energy you put out. Remember, everything is connected. Good comes with the bad. Happiness comes with sadness. So, in moments of unpleasant thoughts, feelings or emotions, find the contrary feeling by digging in a little deeper to find a pleasant aspect. And know that rejection is protection – keep exploring!

Make Yourself Available

Reflective Thought
Let your true self in, to the out.

Mantra
I am available to explore new opportunities for alignment.

Living in Peace
Say "yes" to the invitation

So much happens in a day; it is easy to become unavailable. This isn't only speaking physically – but emotionally and mentally as well. In understanding the essence of slowing down, we can make ourselves available for all that matter. This is not to say that it is necessary to say yes, all the time- nor does it mean making yourself available to all matters, only to what feels right to you. What it means is to be open-minded as unfamiliar arrives along your life path. It is natural to be available for what is familiar. There is a sense of comfort and knowing what to expect. But remember, the bear trap in comfort is that it stagnates growth. The expansion of knowledge from new experiences nourishes growth.

Comfort keeps the space filled with existing and outdated concepts of reality. The space outside of the comfort zone is non- comparable – the space outside of the comfort zone breeds growth. Making yourself available to new opportunities takes a step in the expansive space that holds the unfamiliar new territory to explore. Remember to reflect on this healing journey and take away and apply what tugged closer to you. When making yourself available it is important to practice discernment on distinguishing which opportunities are right for you. Your healing journey will help to sort out what isn't right for you. Trust yourself to decipher as you keep an open mind.

The fear around unfamiliarity can block an open mind and cause a natural gravitation back to comfort. On the contrary, comfort can also protect us from the wrong situations by confirming familiarity of an unpleasant experience. In this instance – remain unavailable. Balance between being available and unavailable by keeping an open mind and staying true to you. The boundaries that you have put in place to protect your energy will support your decision making around your availability. Listen to your inner self.

LIVING IN PEACE

When is the last time you tried something new? It is time to break in some new energy! Say yes to the next invitation or plan a day out with some close ones. Take yourself out for brunch and observe the scenery. Bring in peace, by stepping out of what you are accustomed to. Life has so much to offer and you have just as much to offer life.

Daily Reflection: *When is the last time you tried something new?*

Daily Release: *Release your insecurities verbally and replace with an affirmation. Embrace the new you.*

Unleash Your Growth

Reflective Thought
To grow, I must have space.

Mantra
I am clearing stale energy that no longer has purpose in my life.

Living in Peace
Moment of Self-Reflection

I'd like to connect what I am about to say with the last section, "Make Yourself Available" – growth requires space to truly expand. Several factors can limit a growth mindset by trapping thoughts and restricting the mind from being open, or otherwise, open-minded. Doubt, fear, uncertainty, confusion and skepticism are only a sample of drivers that can prohibit growth from taking place.

Unleash your growth. Know that the more peace you have surrounding you, the quieter the chaos becomes in the background, increasing the chances of reflective decision making that supports a growth mindset. Replace fear with curiosity; doubt with confidence; uncertainty with exploration. Confusion with analysis; and skepticism with optimism.

Focus on transitioning negative thoughts, feelings, emotions and words to those that encourage continued growth. Emotions can be contagious – one negative thought or emotion can easily branch off to multiple negative emotions, suffocating the ability to take a new perspective. That's where being available comes into play. Having an open- mind and being available to new experiences – unleashes growth.

Let's take a step back to three years ago from today. Think back to the goals you made at that time. Cycles you may have closed out since then. Hobbies or interests that were a main part of your life. Now do the same for your current goals, hobbies, etc. What has changed? What is still the same? How does the current version of you align with the older version of you?

Take the moment a step further and pull up a picture of yourself that correlates with the older version of you that you wrote down. Standing in front of the mirror, compare your current self to your old self and recognize the transformation, no matter how subtle or grand. Now take a moment to reflect on what else no longer fits the current version of you and release it, creating space for growth.

LIVING IN PEACE

Grab a piece of paper (no digital devices for this one) and replace a fear you have with the curiosity to understand. Replace a doubt with a confident affirmation; replace a lingering uncertainty with a way to explore it. Replace a sense of confusion with grounded analysis. Replace a skeptical feeling with an optimistic outlook. Come back to this piece of paper at least weekly until each replacement has been met.

Daily Reflection: *Are you holding on to any outdated realities?*

Daily Release: *Release any lingering realities that are creating background noise.*

Emotional Regulation

Reflective Thought

My emotions do not control me. I accept the emotion and embrace how it makes me feel.

Mantra

I address what is in my power to control. Otherwise, I remain unbothered.

Living in Peace

Back to the foundation, take a breather – our breathing holds power!

Emotional regulation is having power and control over our actions when our emotions are coming in hot. It doesn't necessarily mean all the emotions are negative; it could be a mixed bag of emotions from happy to sad and anything in between. But there may be multiple emotions coming in at once. Over stimulating your subconscious – triggering an emotional response. What counts is how you respond both internally AND externally

Often, the focus is our external response; however, internal is equally important. Why? Because holding on to unwanted emotions can open the channel for an unfavorable emotional response. Being self-aware helps recognize the emotion and determine the type of emotion (happy, sad, etc.). Now you accept the emotion, which is usually the step that is overlooked. It is easier to turn a blind eye in hopes the emotion will pass; however, that leaves unsettled or unresolved matters on the table versus addressing the emotion point in time. Once you acknowledge and accept a regulated response comes naturally. A response that is not based on impulse because you allowed yourself to regulate first.

Step into your power and in doing so, you have full power over your emotions. Not the other way around.

Impulsive responses indicate the person, or situation has emotional power over you. So who has power over you? Practice emotional regulation by taking a healthy approach to closing out emotional cycles and fully going through the emotions. Do not rush it. Experience the flow of emotions and process what you are feeling.

Processing is one of the most important steps. Scenario time! Let's say you do not fully process your feelings and emotions, and a trigger strikes your nervous system. Naturally, your emotional side of the brain goes back to the last space you were in, along with the last energy you were in. When your emotions are regulated, your response is guided with the right intention behind it.

Please understand that sometimes an outburst of our emotions is just that, getting out something that needed to come out. That happens from time to time and that is ok. Emotional regulation is not about always standing strong without any emotional reaction. Emotional regulation is about being in control of your emotions and your emotional reaction. If you have an emotional outburst, at the conclusion, bring yourself together and confront the trigger, taking your power back from the trigger.

Battling triggers come with ego deaths. You must submit to the root cause of the trigger no matter the discomfort of addressing it. Most often, triggers are a result of fear or pain – either way, addressing a trigger is likely to bring about unpleasant feelings. Remember, there is no good without bad. The good in addressing a trigger, the trigger loses its power over you and is no longer a trigger. You win!

LIVING IN PEACE

What are your triggers? Take a moment to think of some of the general triggers you have and very specific triggers that surface in specific environments or around certain individuals. As you compare the general trigger to the specific trigger, note your emotional response to each. How does your mood shift? Do you start to visualize a specific incident? These are the emotional triggers to address. This requires more conscious effort. A helpful tip is to go back to the basics with our breathing technique. As you inhale, replace the trigger with a feeling of pleasure or joy. As you release your breath, release the trigger. Overtime, self-regulation will naturally set in, and should the trigger surface, you can regulate your emotional response. If you find it challenging to fully release, work through one emotion at a time if there are multiple and take your time with each one. Some emotions are stronger and take more time to massage out.

Daily Reflection: *How often do you pause and process your emotions before responding?*

Daily Release: *Release the triggers. One at a time.*

Unleash Your Growth

Reflective Thought
Perfection suppresses my natural way of being.

Mantra
I am perfectly unique.

Living in Peace
Connect with nature

The illusion around perfection leads a belief that mistakes are greater in negativity – but a simple tweak of perspective shines light on mistakes being lessons. Lessons that teach us how to handle life. Lessons that are guiding stones to step into alignment of your path. Lessons of breadcrumbs to show how far you've come – the first crumb nowhere in sight. Lessons that are fading into scars – testament to the battles you've overcome.

There is no validity in perfection only social norms that boxes your uniqueness – restricting your individuality from walking your path, in your shoes, at your pace. It is unspoken law that the balance between peace in socialism and peace in solitude is the ultimate form of peace. You have peace both internal and external. You live in peace.

You learn that having people around you, does not me you will not be lonely. We are human – connection is very real. However, if you must alter your way of being – the natural you – your inner spirit, to join in the company of others, you'll never find peace. You are misaligned with self. Knowing what, who, or where to release from nurtures your growth and emotional regulation. What no longer works, it's ok to release it.

That feeling of hesitation, the lump in your throat, the sweaty palms, the racing thoughts. It is all ok. Releasing only allows room for what belongs but does not have room.

Peace in solitude opens your mind and heart to receive what is meant for you, while helping regulate all the feelings that arise. Take a moment to recharge your battery so you do not find yourself alone in a room filled with familiar faces – empty, lost, and untrue to self. Move with grace. Move in truth. Move in awareness to self. Inner peace is the bridge to love. Love is the glue that brings it all in for prosperity and abundance to thrive. Peace in solitude. Love in socialism. Now it's time to explore life from a new perspective. Continuing your path with an update to your journey. Embrace the exploration of the inner YOU.

LIVING IN PEACE

Nature is bountiful. Endless. Powerful. Invigorating. Nature provides, creates, destroys, nurtures, but most of all, nature is love. Spend some time in nature – whatever that looks like for you. Maybe a weekly walk to the park. Gardening. Even dancing in the rain (one of personal favorites). Feel the peace. Set yourself ***FREE.***

Daily Reflection: *Have you made a bucket list? Scratch any off lately?*

Daily Release: *Here is your "free space" to release whatever is calling to you most to release at this very moment.*

PARTING WITH PEACE

This journey started with taking a breath. Do you recall the very first "Moment of Peace"? Learning how to breath all over again. But in a way that brings peace to your nervous system. Now here you are strong in self, aware of your inner power, boundaries established to protect your energy as you continue to show up for you. Remember love, peace, happiness all starts from within – others can only supplement what already exists within you. I'd like to leave you with a special message - healing is a journey. Sometimes a journey we run from because the familiar zone feels too safe, too cozy, too welcoming. The journey can be long years or it could be short. No matter how far you run or how long it takes until your healing is complete, you'll never truly be, **FREE.**

Know that you are loved.

I found gratitude to be a precious and eye-opening part of my healing journey. I challenge you to 30 days of gratitude. To balance what is coming in, I simultaneously challenge you to 30 days of release. The next 30 pages offers space to note your thoughts of gratitude and release what no longer serves you.

Peace, Love & Prosperity

30-day Challenge
Gratitude & Release

Morning Gratitude: Before you start your day, jot down something you are grateful for. If you start feeling troubled or sad throughout the day, come back to this moment of gratefulness.

____

____

____

____

____

____

____

____

End of day Reflection: Good, bad, happy, or sad, what had the greatest impact on your emotions today? Is it an emotion you want to embrace or release?

____

____

____

____

____

____

____

____

Morning Gratitude: Before you start your day, jot down something you are grateful for. If you start feeling troubled or sad throughout the day, come back to this moment of gratefulness.

End of day Reflection: Good, bad, happy, or sad, what had the greatest impact on your emotions today? Is it an emotion you want to embrace or release?

Morning Gratitude: Before you start your day, jot down something you are grateful for. If you start feeling troubled or sad throughout the day, come back to this moment of gratefulness.

End of day Reflection: Good, bad, happy, or sad, what had the greatest impact on your emotions today? Is it an emotion you want to embrace or release?

Morning Gratitude: Before you start your day, jot down something you are grateful for. If you start feeling troubled or sad throughout the day, come back to this moment of gratefulness.

End of day Reflection: Good, bad, happy, or sad, what had the greatest impact on your emotions today? Is it an emotion you want to embrace or release?

Morning Gratitude: Before you start your day, jot down something you are grateful for. If you start feeling troubled or sad throughout the day, come back to this moment of gratefulness.

End of day Reflection: Good, bad, happy, or sad, what had the greatest impact on your emotions today? Is it an emotion you want to embrace or release?

Morning Gratitude: Before you start your day, jot down something you are grateful for. If you start feeling troubled or sad throughout the day, come back to this moment of gratefulness.

____

____

____

____

____

____

____

____

End of day Reflection: Good, bad, happy, or sad, what had the greatest impact on your emotions today? Is it an emotion you want to embrace or release?

____

____

____

____

____

____

____

____

Morning Gratitude: Before you start your day, jot down something you are grateful for. If you start feeling troubled or sad throughout the day, come back to this moment of gratefulness.

End of day Reflection: Good, bad, happy, or sad, what had the greatest impact on your emotions today? Is it an emotion you want to embrace or release?

Morning Gratitude: Before you start your day, jot down something you are grateful for. If you start feeling troubled or sad throughout the day, come back to this moment of gratefulness.

____

End of day Reflection: Good, bad, happy, or sad, what had the greatest impact on your emotions today? Is it an emotion you want to embrace or release?

Morning Gratitude: Before you start your day, jot down something you are grateful for. If you start feeling troubled or sad throughout the day, come back to this moment of gratefulness.

End of day Reflection: Good, bad, happy, or sad, what had the greatest impact on your emotions today? Is it an emotion you want to embrace or release?

Morning Gratitude: Before you start your day, jot down something you are grateful for. If you start feeling troubled or sad throughout the day, come back to this moment of gratefulness.

End of day Reflection: Good, bad, happy, or sad, what had the greatest impact on your emotions today? Is it an emotion you want to embrace or release?

Morning Gratitude: Before you start your day, jot down something you are grateful for. If you start feeling troubled or sad throughout the day, come back to this moment of gratefulness.

End of day Reflection: Good, bad, happy, or sad, what had the greatest impact on your emotions today? Is it an emotion you want to embrace or release?

Morning Gratitude: Before you start your day, jot down something you are grateful for. If you start feeling troubled or sad throughout the day, come back to this moment of gratefulness.

____

____

____

____

____

____

____

____

End of day Reflection: Good, bad, happy, or sad, what had the greatest impact on your emotions today? Is it an emotion you want to embrace or release?

____

____

____

____

____

____

____

____

Morning Gratitude: Before you start your day, jot down something you are grateful for. If you start feeling troubled or sad throughout the day, come back to this moment of gratefulness.

____

End of day Reflection: Good, bad, happy, or sad, what had the greatest impact on your emotions today? Is it an emotion you want to embrace or release?

Morning Gratitude: Before you start your day, jot down something you are grateful for. If you start feeling troubled or sad throughout the day, come back to this moment of gratefulness.

____

____

____

____

____

____

____

____

End of day Reflection: Good, bad, happy, or sad, what had the greatest impact on your emotions today? Is it an emotion you want to embrace or release?

____

____

____

____

____

____

____

____

Morning Gratitude: Before you start your day, jot down something you are grateful for. If you start feeling troubled or sad throughout the day, come back to this moment of gratefulness.

End of day Reflection: Good, bad, happy, or sad, what had the greatest impact on your emotions today? Is it an emotion you want to embrace or release?

Morning Gratitude: Before you start your day, jot down something you are grateful for. If you start feeling troubled or sad throughout the day, come back to this moment of gratefulness.

____

End of day Reflection: Good, bad, happy, or sad, what had the greatest impact on your emotions today? Is it an emotion you want to embrace or release?

Morning Gratitude: Before you start your day, jot down something you are grateful for. If you start feeling troubled or sad throughout the day, come back to this moment of gratefulness.

End of day Reflection: Good, bad, happy, or sad, what had the greatest impact on your emotions today? Is it an emotion you want to embrace or release?

Morning Gratitude: Before you start your day, jot down something you are grateful for. If you start feeling troubled or sad throughout the day, come back to this moment of gratefulness.

____

____

____

____

____

____

____

____

End of day Reflection: Good, bad, happy, or sad, what had the greatest impact on your emotions today? Is it an emotion you want to embrace or release?

____

____

____

____

____

____

____

____

Morning Gratitude: Before you start your day, jot down something you are grateful for. If you start feeling troubled or sad throughout the day, come back to this moment of gratefulness.

____

____

____

____

____

____

____

____

End of day Reflection: Good, bad, happy, or sad, what had the greatest impact on your emotions today? Is it an emotion you want to embrace or release?

____

____

____

____

____

____

____

____

Morning Gratitude: Before you start your day, jot down something you are grateful for. If you start feeling troubled or sad throughout the day, come back to this moment of gratefulness.

____

____

____

____

____

____

____

____

End of day Reflection: Good, bad, happy, or sad, what had the greatest impact on your emotions today? Is it an emotion you want to embrace or release?

____

____

____

____

____

____

____

____

Morning Gratitude: Before you start your day, jot down something you are grateful for. If you start feeling troubled or sad throughout the day, come back to this moment of gratefulness.

____

____

____

____

____

____

____

____

End of day Reflection: Good, bad, happy, or sad, what had the greatest impact on your emotions today? Is it an emotion you want to embrace or release?

____

____

____

____

____

____

____

____

Morning Gratitude: Before you start your day, jot down something you are grateful for. If you start feeling troubled or sad throughout the day, come back to this moment of gratefulness.

End of day Reflection: Good, bad, happy, or sad, what had the greatest impact on your emotions today? Is it an emotion you want to embrace or release?

Morning Gratitude: Before you start your day, jot down something you are grateful for. If you start feeling troubled or sad throughout the day, come back to this moment of gratefulness.

____

____

____

____

____

____

____

____

End of day Reflection: Good, bad, happy, or sad, what had the greatest impact on your emotions today? Is it an emotion you want to embrace or release?

____

____

____

____

____

____

____

____

Morning Gratitude: Before you start your day, jot down something you are grateful for. If you start feeling troubled or sad throughout the day, come back to this moment of gratefulness.

____

End of day Reflection: Good, bad, happy, or sad, what had the greatest impact on your emotions today? Is it an emotion you want to embrace or release?

Morning Gratitude: Before you start your day, jot down something you are grateful for. If you start feeling troubled or sad throughout the day, come back to this moment of gratefulness.

____

____

____

____

____

____

____

____

End of day Reflection: Good, bad, happy, or sad, what had the greatest impact on your emotions today? Is it an emotion you want to embrace or release?

____

____

____

____

____

____

____

____

Morning Gratitude: Before you start your day, jot down something you are grateful for. If you start feeling troubled or sad throughout the day, come back to this moment of gratefulness.

End of day Reflection: Good, bad, happy, or sad, what had the greatest impact on your emotions today? Is it an emotion you want to embrace or release?

Morning Gratitude: Before you start your day, jot down something you are grateful for. If you start feeling troubled or sad throughout the day, come back to this moment of gratefulness.

End of day Reflection: Good, bad, happy, or sad, what had the greatest impact on your emotions today? Is it an emotion you want to embrace or release?

Morning Gratitude: Before you start your day, jot down something you are grateful for. If you start feeling troubled or sad throughout the day, come back to this moment of gratefulness.

End of day Reflection: Good, bad, happy, or sad, what had the greatest impact on your emotions today? Is it an emotion you want to embrace or release?

Morning Gratitude: Before you start your day, jot down something you are grateful for. If you start feeling troubled or sad throughout the day, come back to this moment of gratefulness.

____

____

____

____

____

____

____

____

End of day Reflection: Good, bad, happy, or sad, what had the greatest impact on your emotions today? Is it an emotion you want to embrace or release?

____

____

____

____

____

____

____

____

Morning Gratitude: Before you start your day, jot down something you are grateful for. If you start feeling troubled or sad throughout the day, come back to this moment of gratefulness.

End of day Reflection: Good, bad, happy, or sad, what had the greatest impact on your emotions today? Is it an emotion you want to embrace or release?

www.ingramcontent.com/pod-product-compliance
Lightning Source LLC
LaVergne TN
LVHW050539100826
845148LV00002B/613

* 9 7 9 8 2 3 4 0 2 7 3 7 5 *